CLEANING EAR WAX GUIDE

~~~

By Emily Taylor
~~~

The information herein is offered for informational purposes solely, and is universal as so. The presentation of the information is without contract or any type of guarantee assurance.

The trademarks that are used are without any consent, and the publication of the trademark is without permission or backing by the trademark owner. All trademarks and brands within this book are for clarifying purposes only and are the owned by the owners themselves, not affiliated with this document.

TABLE OF CONTENTS

ALL ABOUT EARWAX REMOVAL: BREAKING DOWN THE ESSENTIALS, MYTHS, AND CONCEPTS

Ears are a very important part of the body. They are responsible for having the ability to hear. This is why it is crucial to give extra care for your ears. In addition, the internal parts of the ear are known to be quite sensitive.

The good news is, there are plenty of safe ways to clean your ear that even a doctor would suggest doing. You would also learn about unconventional methods such as ear candling.

Sadly, myths and misconceptions about ear cleaning abound, and some people fall victim to these. Plenty of cases are reported in which people get involved in incidents that cause damage to their hearing, may it be temporary or permanent. Some of these incidents involve improper cleaning.

This is why we need to be educated on the topic before considering engaging in any measure to cure ear related problems that might have occurred through diseases or through mishandling of the ears.

In this guide, you will be able to learn more about the human ear. Understanding its parts and functions is key to highlighting the importance of treating it with care. You will also learn how to clean it properly and also, learn about what may be the reasons for the appearance and look of your earwax. You will also know about some of the more common myths about ears, particularly about cleaning them.

Armed with this information, you will finally get to make a wise decision which method of ear cleaning would work the best for you.

If you are unsure on what method is the most appropriate for you, then you'll be glad to know that we'll be sharing information regarding exactly that.

I hope you enjoy this and learn lots of amazing facts about the organ that's responsible for allowing you to enjoy sound.

WHAT IS EARWAX?

Earwax is a waxy secretion from the ears of both humans and mammals. It may be waxy in texture, but it is not literally wax.

It is the glands of the external ear which secrete this yellowish substance, the medical term for which is cerumen. It can be used interchangeably with the word 'earwax'. However, the substance that we usually observe in our ears is usually a mixture of oil and sweat as well as cerumen.

Its color can range from gray, to orange and even yellow. These colors may vary for plenty of reasons such as genetics, how stressed you have been feeling, your environment or the amount of dirt that may have entered your ear, and other diseases with symptoms that affect the color and texture of your earwax.

Now, all of us know that hygiene comes with thorough cleaning of the body including the parts which are oftentimes ignored such as the inside of our belly button, nose and, the ear.

These areas can be characterized by certain smells which are brought by the buildup of dirt and bacteria. For example, the belly button stores lint and sweat, and our nose filters the air we breathe, accumulating unpleasant yet minute substances, while in the ears, there is buildup of oil and dead skin cells). Earwax may also come with a certain smell which may be caused by bacteria.

WHY IS EARWAX IMPORTANT?

It is important to understand our body and every little thing could contribute to our health. Earwax is part of how our human body functions, so it's crucial that we know the

With this being stated, is earwax something we should clean regularly? Or is it okay to just shrug off and clean whenever we just feel like it. To tell you the truth, earwax are actually a very healthy production of our body!

The cerumen serves as a lining to our ears. Thanks to this substance, our ears are naturally provided with lubrication, and surprisingly, protection from bacteria! What people say about earwax – that it is bad and unhygienic -- is actually a misconception!

Earwax has a purpose, which is to protect the human ear from things like dust, dirt, insects, water, and other foreign objects that may pass through the ear canal. It serves as lubrication to the ear canal and is also helpful in fighting off any bacteria that may cause complications in the ear.

It is true that having too much earwax can be a huge health risk to humans but what people seem to forget is the fact that having too little earwax is very dangerous as well. This is because if you do not have a sufficient amount of earwax present, you are more susceptible to ear infections, and tiny things like bugs and dirt can go straight into your eardrum, causing damage manifested in hearing loss.

DO WE REALLY NEED TO REMOVE EARWAX?

Yes, earwax removal is necessary in certain cases. While too little of something can be harmful, the same thing applies when there's too much. That's why we still have to remove earwax when it becomes too much.

Too much earwax can cause health risks such as vertigo. Earwax blocks the eardrums, and if the ear is impacted with this substance, you will experience difficulty hearing. There will also be too much pressure in your inner ears, which can be uncomfortable. Also, the body's ability to balance itself will be more difficult.

Another health risk also includes tinnitus. Causes of tinnitus include: prolonged exposure to very loud sounds, whether it is through earphones or regular speakers and also, earwax stuck in the ear.

Having too much ear wax can also result to ear ache, ear infection, and ear itchiness. This is why it's very important to clean your ears when needed, just make sure you do not overdo it.

EARWAX:
HISTORY AND SCIENCE

There have been researches about how earwax has the ability to track down your ancestry. It has been observed that among people of African descent and those who are of European descent, earwax secretions tend to be described as more pungent or foul smelling, when compared to those from people from the East of Asia and, also some from the Native America. So to put it simply, your race may have an effect on what your earwax looks and smells like.

This brings us to a quite peculiar topic. There have been a few researches stating that people with white and dryer earwax tend to have less body odor as opposed to people with darker yellow and stinky earwax.

Several generations back, people from East Asia have similar traits as other races when it comes to the earwax production. However, East Asians developed mutations in their genes, and these were passed on to the current generation.

People residing in areas around East Asia now have lack certain chemicals that make up body odor. This is because of their ABCC11 gene. This specific gene is the one in charge of determining whether the ear wax is dry or wet and is also responsible for having body odor.

The fact that earwax has such a pungent scent is one of the reasons that people believe it is unsanitary. But science shows otherwise. So if your earwax seems to be a darker color or has a strong scent, it doesn't mean that you are unhygienic or unhealthy.

In the highly popular book "The American Frugal Housewife" by Lydia Maria Francis Child, it has been stated that earwax is used to heal small wounds (specifically ones caused by skewers, nails and etc.) as it does, in fact, has anti-bacterial properties. It has been said in the book that it should be applied as soon as possible to minimize pain. It can act also act an old-fashioned lip balm or lip salve to help with chapped lips.

Some people back then are believed to have used earwax because of its many purposes and benefits. The notion is still unpleasant for many people though, so it's fortunate that alternatives have been developed and they can be just as effective. We can buy different ointments and lip balms in the store instead of using what is basically a mixture of our sweat, cells, and oils!

History can be very amusing for sure. Manuscripts were usually written with ink that some of the ink contained earwax. Well of course, humans evolve, gain more intelligence and resources each and every day, which is why this is no longer in practice. However, in the past, people have no choice but to use things that most people may consider strange when used today.

Some earwax cleaning methods also used to be popular methods but advances in science and medicine proved them to be harmful. One particular example is syringing. This method isn't done as much as it was years ago because several complications have been reported to come with it. This method is not only said to be ineffective in cleaning earwax build-up; it has also been proven to increase the risk of ear infections. This is the exact opposite of what we want to happen.

WHAT YOUR EARWAX SAYS ABOUT YOU: IS IT NORMAL OR IS IT A PROBLEM?

Ear wax varies from person to person. Certain characteristics of your earwax may indicate whether it's normal or that you have a medical condition that you need to take care of.

As stated earlier, your genes may affect the consistency and odor of your earwax, but what part of that range is considered normal? What are the signs to look out for before consulting your doctor? These questions will be answered in this section. The physical attributes of your earwax and texture may reveal interesting things about your health.

YELLOW, MOIST, AND STICKY

This type of earwax is very common in adults. Earwax normally feels like this because it serves as a natural lubrication for your ear to keep it from becoming dry and itchy. If you observe your earwax to be like this, then it's a sign that you're normal and healthy.

DARK AND STICKY EARWAX

This color of earwax is also perfectly healthy although it's understandable why people are concerned when they observe that they have this kind of earwax. People who possess this type of earwax also usually have strong body odor due to a chemical present in their sweat. This is nothing to worry about and is all related to ones genetics.

LIGHT YELLOW EARWAX

While adults usually have a more saturated hue of yellow in their ears, children are most likely to have lighter-colored earwax. The reason for this is because younger people tend to produce a lot more earwax than older people. The reason why the color of their earwax is paler is that it gets removed quickly and is immediately replaced with newer, lighter colored, earwax.

GRAY EARWAX

This color may seem odd to some because earwax is known for its yellow hues, but having this shade come out of your ear exhibits that your earwax is doing what it's meant to do: collect anything that may pass through your ear canal and protect your eardrum! The gray color is from the dirt that may have gathered over time. This is totally normal unless the consistency of this earwax is dry and flaky.

Having dry, flaky, and gray/white earwax may be a sign that you are suffering from seborrheic eczema. This condition will manifest in areas where skin is most often oily. If you have these symptoms, it may be a good idea to go visit your doctor so that you can receive treatments for this condition.

THICK AND DARK EARWAX

When you are under so much stress and anxiety, your body tends to produce more earwax than usual. This is due to your body perspiring a lot more than usual when put into situations that can lead to such emotions. This may be a sign that you need to relax yourself due to the harsh effects extreme stress do to you in the long run. While being under constant stress isn't something considered good for your body and can even cause serious damage if not taken care of, it means that your body is responding properly to certain circumstances that may have been very useful for survival.

BLACK OR EXTREMELY DARK BROWN

Extremely dark wax is quite a frightening sight to see, but this is also nothing to worry about. This shade is usually caused by the overproduction of earwax due to stress. The black/dark brown color may also be the result of the cerumen staying in the ear for longer. Exposure to oxygen can cause the wax to darken.

WET AND RUNNY EAR WAX

Having small amounts earwax leaking from your ears is normal. This means your ears are cleaning itself out of the excess earwax inside your ear; this is a totally natural process. The time when you should worry is when the leakage is excessive, has pus or traces of blood. These are signs of having a ruptured eardrum. In this case, immediately see a doctor to seek medical treatment for any damage in your ear that may cause temporary or permanent hearing loss.

BLOODY EARWAX

It's scary to see blood come out of your ear. Older people tend to have earwax that may be similar to this color because they produce a lot less earwax than younger people. Other than that, traces of blood in your earwax can be caused by having a ruptured eardrum or even something even more serious such as cancer.

WHY IT IS IMPORTANT TO CLEAN YOUR EARS SAFELY

As you have read, earwax is essential in keeping our ears protected. Nonetheless, it isn't uncommon for people to go and try to clean their ears and remove earwax. In fact, many of us were taught that regular cleaning of the ears—specifically the ear canal—is required so that we can remain hygienic. However, this is not always true. Earwax should only be removed when there's too much.

Did you know that the most common cause of ear blockage is from cleaning it with things such as cotton swabs, hair pins, and other sharp foreign objects that may be inserted into the ear canal? This is something that plenty of experts have advised against, but has been done anyway because people like to think that they are clean and hygienic. There's also the fact that it has been universally practiced for so long.

The reason why it is so harmful is that these objects are more likely to push back the excess wax into your ear when it should have already been released from your ear naturally. This creates a large build-up of the secretion.

You may use proper cleaning implements such as cotton swabs but even they should not be used further than the entrance of the ear. Keep in mind that they are for external use only.

Improper cleaning of the ears is one factor that may cause this blockage. However, blockage can also naturally occur in people who were born with small ear canals that make it harder for their ears to keep themselves clean on their own. One of the conditions that may cause people to have an abnormally small ear canal is called "Microtia" and is caused by a gene abnormality.

This makes people prone to ear infections. If you have Microtia, it is especially important that you regularly clean your ears in order to avoid blockage.

So, what if you are not born with any defect in your genes that may require you to constantly clean out your ears of any remaining debris, do you still need to clean your ears?

Well, the answer varies depending on how you clean your ears and what methods you use to do it. Most people clean their ears with improper materials and tend to do it quite harshly. When you clean your ears with proper devices, solutions and, do it in moderation, you are not likely to disrupt the natural production of this waxy protective substance. There have been thousands of cases—in children alone—wherein their eardrums have been damaged from attempts on cleaning their ears improperly.

Cleaning your ears is a satisfying feeling, seeing all the wax being removed can make a person feel like they are being hygienic, but the truth is, using the wrong methods can worsen the current state of your ears. Your ears are a very sensitive part of your body and one wrong move can easily cause serious injuries and even permanent hearing loss.

HOW TO SAFELY CLEAN YOUR EARS

When people clean their ears, many do the common mistake of going in too deep their ear canal causing injuries to thousands of people who attempt this.

So, how do we clean our ears without damaging it?

USE COTTON SWABS PROPERLY

Well, this may sound surprising, but don't use a cotton swab inside your ear! If you look at the labels in most brands that sell cotton swabs, it clearly says "for external use only." There is absolutely no reason to use it to clean your inner ear? This should only be used for cleaning the outer parts of the ear.

The only time it is appropriate to use cotton swabs is when you are only cleaning the external parts or areas close to the opening of your ear. Going any deeper into your ear can be quite risky. A small abrasion in your ear is an easy way to get a nasty infection since the inside of your ear is naturally moist which the perfect breeding ground for different types of bacteria.

BE GENTLE

Always keep in mind that you should be careful with what you use in your ear. Cleaning it must be a gentle process. People should always remember that ear cleaning shouldn't be done aggressively. It's not uncommon for people to use Q-tips, or even hair pins (yes, hair pins!) inside their ear. There are numerous complications that can lead to having foreign, sharp objects inside your ear, one of this called Otitis Externa or most commonly referred to as Swimmer's Ear.

This is the infection of the skin that is caused by different kinds of bacteria namely streptococcus or pseudomonas. It is caused by skin disorders such as eczema or dermatitis, but swimmer's ear can also be caused by mishandling of things such as sand, cotton swabs or, any other sharp objects and even accidentally putting shampoo inside the ear canal or submerging your head in a bubble bath or any body of water (thus the name Swimmer's Ear)

Early signs of this certain infection include itchiness and the sensation of clogging; swelling shows up as a later symptom alongside ear pain. There are plenty of treatments for this such as using antibacterial ear drops (may this have steroids or not) or pain relievers. But like what they always say, prevention is always much better than cure.

LET PROFESSIONALS HANDLE IT

Anything long enough to go past your ear canal and into your eardrum should never be handled by someone who does not have medical knowledge about the ear.

ONLY CLEAN EARWAX WHEN THERE'S TOO MUCH

You should also always keep in mind that you should only clean up only the excess earwax build-up you may have in your ear. Any more wax found deep inside the ear canal should be left unless it has become jammed inside your ear and has been affecting your ears negatively

There are plenty of other methods that are best suited for the internal cleaning of the ear such as using something such as ear wax softeners or using a special device to irrigate your ears are very common remedies to impacted ears, even homemade remedies are available in your own kitchen that is just as safe. What's important is that you carefully follow the instructions given to you whenever you attempt to clean your ears.

COMMON MISCONCEPTIONS

Myth #1: Earwax is unhygienic

One of the most common misconceptions about earwax is that it is unhygienic and unsanitary, and that you need to have it regularly removed and cleaned.

While excess earwax build-up can be quite harmful and even painful, people always tend to rigorously clean it.

It is healthy to produce earwax. Earwax is important to protect the eardrum. If you think that earwax would get stuck overtime if you do not clean it out as soon as you possibly can, then what you have been led to believe is wrong. So long as your jaw is active, moving or overall, working the way it should (may it be in terms of chewing or anything similar to this), the earwax will eventually make its way out of the ear with all the small specs of dirt, germs and, microorganisms that may have made its way to your ear.

Myth #2: Using cotton swabs is always safe

Cotton swabs are something people use on a regular basis. Seeing the bright-yellow residue on the swab leads people to believe that you really are cleaning your ears, but this is untrue!

Whenever you clean your ears with a cotton swab, you are pushing the earwax further towards your eardrums, the reason why we see the yellowish deposit is because the earwax naturally pushes itself out from the body, whenever ears get wet or moistened this means your ears are cleaning itself naturally, very similar to cat!

Misuse of cotton swabs is actually the leading cause of having buildups in your ear. Other things not meant for your ear such as hair pins, matches, and your own nails can cause abrasions within the ear canal and cause an infection. Though ear infections are extremely painful, there are plenty of treatments that your doctor may prescribe to aid in curing these complications.

Myth #3: We have to religiously clean our ears.

It does not matter if you use the proper materials the clean out your ears, earwax softening drops, homemade remedies, ear cleaning kits, you name it!—*over cleaning is over cleaning*—so it is very essential to give your ears time to produce the needed earwax and only clean it whenever there is any excess or if your ENT says so. Always let a skilled practitioner do the job for you when dealing with much more serious ear related problems!

Myth #4: Children always get ear infection due to earwax.

The thing is, children usually get ear complications is to the fact that their mothers try to clean their ears too often for hygienic reasons. This is bad practice.

Cleaning ears far too often may cause the child to get dirt inside their ears and consequently risk developing nasty ear complications such as infections and having bits of cotton getting stuck inside their ear.

If you do not know yet, ear infections most commonly affect children. The reason this occurs more often to children is that the tubes connecting the middle ear to the back of the nose (scientifically referred to as the Eustachian Tube) don't function as well as it does to older people.

Younger children's Eustachian tubes haven't developed yet and are somewhat more horizontal, smaller, flatter, and shorter than what adults have. Otitis media or the infection of the middle has the common symptoms of earache. This happens when infants are in distress because of things such as blocked nasal passages from colds, but this condition is not limited to younger people, adults may have this as well if they do not care for their ears properly.

Ear infections do not usually last for that long, but when it happens, it is usually extremely painful and unpleasant for the ones suffering from it. When it lasts longer than expected, it may be a sign of something more serious within your body. The

Eustachian tubes of children usually improve when they have reached the age of 7.

Myth #5 Itchy ears and other ear problems are frequently caused by earwax.

Whenever your ears are slightly itchy or if you're experiencing slight loss of hearing, many people assume that the cause of it is excess buildup of earwax. People have to always keep in mind that there are plenty of other reasons why you're experiencing these symptoms.

If ever you feel like you are experiencing these symptoms, do not do things to your ear on your own unless you are sure that it is from any excess buildup that may have accumulated. Water inside of your ear can rupture your ear and worsen your condition.

In the next section, you will learn more about the more common ear complications. You will also learn about the conditions in which earwax and its removal will have an important role.

EAR COMPLICATIONS AND TREATMENTS

Upon feeling discomfort in their ears, some people think that the earwax is to blame and immediately try to clean their ears with earwax softeners, cotton swabs, and other treatments that may be bought in the store. While an impacted ear may be causing any of the symptoms one may be feeling, well, that isn't always the case.

There are plenty of other possible complications that may affect your ear that isn't due to excess earwax, so don't go grabbing your cotton swabs and poke it into your ear! Here are the different complications and the treatments for it. If you are experiencing the symptoms of these complications, go book an appointment with your doctor.

WHAT TO EXPECT WHEN GETTING DIAGNOSED

The doctors should have a clear view of what the condition of the eardrum is due to the fact that many illnesses that show symptoms in places away from the ear may root from complications in the ear.

Medical professionals use different medical devices such as the otoscope, is an instrument with lightning and magnifying systems used for visual examinations of the tympanic membrane and the canal connecting it to the exterior of the body. This is used to check whether there are impactions, infections or, any type of foreign objects that's shouldn't be in the ear, this is likely to be very common with children who oftentimes have troubles with getting toys or any small object inside their ears (or even nose, mouth and the likes).

Otoscopes are used for many purposes such as checkup for any sort of physical exam. This item is also very useful when it comes to screening any infections amongst babies or children.

BULLOUS MYRINGITIS

This condition is an ear infection wherein blisters that are filled with fluid are present in the internal parts of the ear. This infection can be caused by bacteria that can result to other types of infections as well. This condition can be cured in just a few days.

If you are experiencing symptoms such as severe pain, fever, hearing loss, and excessive leaking from the ear, or discomfort, then you might be suffering from Bullous Myringitis. People who have diseases such as the flu or cold are more prone to contracting this disease.

Doctors may prescribe over the counter medications as well as antibiotics as treatment. The symptoms of the infection may be extremely painful and uncomfortable, but with proper care may subside within the span of 2 days.

OTITIS MEDIA

This is can be a viral or bacterial infection. This condition affects the middle ear. This illness is the second most common type of ear infection in children.

The bacteria or viruses present in the ear causes a build-up of pus and mucus behind the eardrum, thereby blocking the Eustachian tube. Because of this, swelling and pain may occur. Other symptoms may include fever, fatigue, and glue ear. Glue ear is a symptom in which fluids block the middle ear (more on this later). This is referred to as otitis media with effusion.

Most doctors will not prescribe any treatment for this because the swelling will naturally subside within a week. In addition, antibiotics won't always help because they will not speed up the healing process if the infection is caused by a virus. Antibiotics may even result to certain side effects such as diarrhea, rashes, or feeling ill, so doctors try not to recommend taking this.

Painkillers such as Paracetamol or Ibuprofen may be used to alleviate the pain. Of course, if symptoms last longer than usual, this may be a sign of something more serious.

OTITIS EXTERNA

This is also known as Swimmer's Ear. This infection is located at the outer part of the ear canal which is causing it to be red in color and having it swell up. Certain things can cause this such as fungal infections, allergies, and irritation. You may be prone to developing swimmer's ear if you have damaged the skin in the internal part of your ear, if fluid gets into your ear, or if you live in a place where the temperature is high.

This condition is very common in tropical countries. There are a few ways to prevent this condition:

- Wear ear plugs before swimming
- Avoid inserting things deep into your ear canal
- Keep your ears dry at all times.

Oftentimes, the treatment doctor prescribes are ear drops or sprays that contain steroids to tone down the swelling and itchiness.

PERFORATED EARDRUM

This is also known as the, ruptured eardrum. When there is a defect or wound on a thin membrane that divides the ear canal to the middle ear, a perforated eardrum usually occurs. Having this may lead to a significant pain, infection in the middle ear, and even deafness.

One of the main causes of perforated eardrums are injuries (such as head trauma), Otitis Media (also known as Swimmer's Ear: The accumulation of fluid in the ear), Prolonged exposure to loud, noisy sounds (Acoustic Trauma) or, having sharp foreign objects puncture the ear.

Having a perforated eardrum can actually be very inconvenient for many reasons. There are some instances in which a person does not feel the symptoms of it. For example, some people are diagnosed with the said disease can ride a plane without experiencing excruciating pain in their ears. Ear pain is generally experienced due to changes in pressure. The Eustachian tube connects the middle ear to the nose. It has the important role of equalizing the pressure in the middle ear. When going up to higher altitudes, the pressure in the middle ear adjusts to the pressure of the air around you.

If the case of a perforated eardrum is too severe (when the skull is affected), the chances of hearing loss gets higher. But if the case is not as critical, tinnitus or experiencing "ringing" sensations can take place.

This condition has no needed special medication as this usually heals up on its own within the duration of roughly 3 months. There has been no specific medical treatment for this but medical professionals may recommend you to intake antibiotics. This is order to avoid any infection that can be more dangerous and costly in the long run if not treated properly. Having chronic infection through a perforated eardrum can result to temporary or permanent hearing loss.

Although this certain case does not really need any serious medical treatment, there are some situations that the hole or the rupture is too severe that having to undergo surgery is required to avoid any further damage.

After the cause of a ruptured ear, the symptoms usually show up almost immediately. Symptoms such as tinnitus (hearing a ringing sensation), vertigo (spinning sensation) and nausea due to having vertigo, hearing loss, and earache and leakage of pus get into place. Once you have experienced symptoms that are quite similar to the ones above-mentioned, then it is best to see a doctor before the case gets too severe.

A ruptured eardrum is definitely not a pleasant experience at all, but here are ways on how you can prevent this from happening. Of course, having protection from too much loud noise is very important, wearing ear plugs or ear muffs are recommended when extremely loud noises are unavoidable.

Make sure that the volume on your earphones or speakers are not in the maximum setting to avoid long exposure to heavy noise. You may not realize this but having your music on too loud is very dangerous and risky, so try to think about your ears before jamming to your favorite songs.

If you always go to concerts where there is usually loud music, try to get a pair of ear muffs that reduce noise. That way, your ears stay protected.

Next, consider having protection gears for the head when using motorcycles or bikes to avoid any sort of accidents. Be more attentive to your surroundings.

Being careless is one of the most common reasons why people suffer the complications of having a perforated eardrum.

Another thing to remember is to seek help from a doctor whenever any signs are showing. Infections are extremely uncomfortable and can easily occur to anyone.

Lastly, never stick anything through your ears ever. Having any foreign object in your ear, whether sharp or not, can be extremely dangerous to your ears because the eardrum is extremely sensitive.

One common misconception is, if your ears are itchy, it is dirty. As a result, people instinctively scratch their ears with whatever sharp object in order to remove the "dirt" inside their ears. This is a big no-no. If you want your ears cleaned, have it done the right way, whether it is through homemade remedies that has been proven to be safe or through a doctor. Keep in mind that cotton swabs can push your earwax further and can also graze the flesh in the inside of your ear causing it to have abrasions, which can ultimatelyin the end result to a ruptured eardrum or an infection.

GLUE EAR

The middle ear is supposed to be filled mostly with air, but with glue ear your middle ear is blocked with a sticky, glue-like, fluid that can dampen the vibrations of the sound-waves passing through your ear. This can cause people who are suffering from this have troubles in hearing efficiently, which may lead to behavioral problems in younger people.

This condition poses negative psychological effects, specifically in children. When this condition is left unnoticed, children may have difficulty learning in school because they could not understand what the teacher is saying. Consequently, they may have troubles in their behavior because they cannot hear their parents well. This may cause them to feel left out because they couldn't understand what other people are saying, making them quiet. Of course, this case wouldn't be as likely if you are an adult because you would immediately notice that your hearing is somewhat impaired and will immediately seek help.

There are a few indicators for glue ear in children such as:

- Dulled hearing
- problems with social interactions due to speech and hearing problems,
- problems with their balance,
- not being to follow instructions properly,
- propensity to turn up the volume often, and
- being unresponsive to sounds

Always watch out for these signs as these can be easily misunderstood by people as a behavioral problem rather than a physical problem.

One of the major factors that may cause children to suffer from glue ear is having either a very narrow or blocked Eustachian tubes which may mess up the balance of fluid and air inside the ears. A child may develop glue ear if they have caught any common diseases such as the cold or the flu. The excess mucus can make it difficult for the tube to drain out the excess fluid inside the ear.

Specialists have tested different ways to cure glue ear such as antibiotics, decongestants, and steroids. None of these treatments seem to work for people who are suffering from this. Doctors often tell their patients to wait for about 3 months to see if the affected ear has been cleared.

There is another method which can be done wherein the patient regularly blows a balloon with their nose to help open up the Eustachian tube and hopefully drain out the fluid. In severe cases, the glue ear may last for more than usual. This is the time when the doctor would usually recommend the patient to undergo a minor operation, but this isn't often done as most cases of glue ear clear up on its own without the need of any treatment.

While waiting for the symptoms of glue ear to wear down, a child may wear hearing aids to be able to hear properly until the glue ear has cleared. This will only be temporary and will be removed. It is important to speak with a specialist about to because some children may develop anxiety wearing hearing aids regularly.

EUSTACHIAN TUBE BLOCKAGE

Having the cold or the flu that most of us can get from time to time and is also usually accompanied by the feeling of having your ears clogged. This is due to the fluids and mucus getting trapped in your ear instead of flowing down your throat like they naturally should.

Although clogged ears alone aren't usually painful, it can be such an annoying feeling when the sounds we hear are muffled. This usually isn't serious and has happened to all of us when we do things such as riding a plane.

One method that you may try to do to unclog your ears is called the Valsalva maneuver, or as many people like to call it "popping your ears." You can do this by taking a deep breath, pinching your nose, and blowing down on it hard. Once you have done this, the feeling having your ears clogged will usually subside. Steaming is another option too loosens the mucus, or even the use of ear drops and other over the counter medication.

Go see a doctor if you are experiencing more than one symptom in your ear because this may be diagnosed as an illness.

CERUMEN IMPACTION

This is the time when ear cleaning is actually needed. There are plenty of homemade remedies as well as professional services that may work for you to release any excess earwax located inside your ear.

This is quite easy to remove, but leaving it without proper treatment can cause hearing loss, vertigo, tinnitus, and other problems in the ear. This is caused by having a small ear canal or accidentally pushing back the earwax into the ear canal. Further on, you will be able to learn about which methods are worth trying in order to maintain the cleanliness of the ear without causing any form of harm.

HOMEMADE REMEDIES

Not everyone has the time, opportunity and, money to go to a medical professional who specializes in ENT (ear, nose, and throat) or someone who practices earwax removal. While it is very much better to go and seek help from these people, if your goal is to only clean your ears, but have no significantly or relatively risky and dangerous health condition such as what is said above (vertigo, tinnitus, cough, infections, pain and, other ear complications) you can absolutely try natural homemade remedies. Just be very careful in doing so.

Basically, the three main objectives of ear wax removal at home are to soften, to loosen, and to help your ear naturally clean out the excess buildup that may have accumulated through time.

This list will contain things you already have on hand and, you can easily do in the comforts of your home. These homemade solutions has the objective to soften ear wax making it easier to come out of your ear naturally rather than forcing it with the use of cotton swabs, bobby pins, nails and other small objects that should never come close to your ear canal.

THE OLD-FASHIONED GO-TO AMONG MOMS -- THE SALTWATER SOLUTION

Salt contains many antibacterial properties and minerals that can be used to avoid earwax impaction and also prevent serious ear condition—mainly infection.

Saltwater is a light antiseptic and is gentle enough to use around your ear. Not only is this an effective remedy for cleaning your ears, salt water has also been used in helping relieve the symptoms of strep throat or sore throat.

1. Take 1 teaspoon of salt and ½ cup of warm water (the ratio is preferably 1:24 salt to water) take a cotton ball, and soak it in the salt water solution.

2. With your head facing in an upright position, put a few drops of the saltwater using the cotton ball into the ear.

3. Stay in that position for not more than 5 minutes.

TIP: If you have a pipet or a small medicine dropper, you can use this instead of a cotton ball for a much easier application.

EVERYONE'S FAVORITE MOISTURIZER -- BABY OIL

Baby oil or mineral oil is derived from petroleum which is mostly used for the skin, Mineral oil is light, has no scent and also, has no color (clear), and it is very gentle as is it obviously used for babies who naturally have sensitive and delicate skin.

The method of applying baby oil is quite similar to the previous method.

1. Take a few drops of the oil with a medicine dropper, pipet or soaked cotton and put it in the ear.

2. Take a dry cotton ball and put it on top of the ear so the oil (that is now in the ear) does not spill or ooze out.

3. Again, leave this for several minutes. Then, with a soft cloth, clean the outside part of your ear to remove the residue or the excess baby oil.

GOOD FOR YOUR SALAD, GOOD FOR YOUR EARS: OLIVE OIL

Olive oil has anti-bacterial properties that may aid in preventing ear infections. Not only that, it also has the ability to lessen the chances of having any complications with your ears, and help clean it by softening the hard, compacted, earwax.

This method is a fairly quick and easy method to clean your ears, and olive oil is also readily available in your kitchen. This particular method is very similar to using baby oil on your ears.

1. First, warm up a small amount of olive oil, making sure that it is tolerable to touch (you do not want to burn yourself!) You can warm up your oil by putting it in the stove in a very low heat. If you're not really in the mood for heating up a stove, you can use your microwave and put it there for around 10-15 seconds.

2. Next, with a pipet or a medicine dropper, put 3-4 drops of the oil into the ear and allow it to sit for 8-12 minutes before cleaning it all off.

TIP: Coconut oil and mustard oil are good alternatives. They are just as effective.

TRY TO GET YOUR HANDS ON ONE OF THESE: ELEPHANT EAR WASHERS!

If you live in a household with a relatively big family, and hygiene is your number one priority, try to get one of these elephant ear washers.

What this basically does is irrigate your ears. They loosen up the earwax buildup with a very gentle pressure from the warm water.

The earwax is drained from your ear into a small basin or canister. This very easy practice is used by families who are short on their budget since visiting medical professionals can't be afforded by some and can also be quite pricey. Irrigation is a method that professionals usually offer whenever

HYDROGEN PEROXIDE

This bleaching agent is commonly found in first aid kits because it is an effective cleaning agent. Hydrogen peroxide can be found in almost every household especially to the people with little ones who like to go outside for a playtime and goes home with an ouchie on their knee. Hydrogen peroxide is a very effective disinfectant and cleanser and without a doubt, you can use this for ears as well!

To use this, simply add a few drops of hydrogen peroxide in your ear with a pipet or a medicine dropper; fill your ear up until you see the hydrogen peroxide fizz or, bubble.

Keep this in your ear and maintain your head in a still position to prevent spilling, do this for about 5 minutes only and make sure to not overdo it. Clean or blot your ears with a tissue or a towel until you feel the outer part dry. Repeat this process in the other ear and you are done! What this does is soften your earwax, which is handy especially when it is impacted or is located way inside your ear canal.

VINEGAR AND RUBBING ALCOHOL

People who remove earwax at home have found that these two ingredients when combined are the most effective. These two have been used for decades as a multipurpose, natural cleanser.

Vinegar is well known to be an effective ingredient used for cooking to preserve and to avoid spoilage; vinegar is also used for household cleaning specifically for molds, moss and foul odors. Also, did you know that vinegar is good for internal use? Specific types of vinegar such as apple cider can be great for the skin and also for weight management. For the ear, vinegar acts as an anti-bacterial and anti-fungal agent.

Rubbing alcohol in the other hand is responsible for drying and evaporating the earwax, which is helpful if your goal is to get rid of some.

1. To use this, simply mix a 1:1 ratio of vinegar and alcohol. Do not use more than a tablespoon of each ingredient since you don't need too much

2. Using a dropper or a cotton ball submerged in the said solution, take about 3-4 drops in your ear (which is now supposed to be titled up).

3. Stay still for about 3-5 minutes so that the wax has time to loosen up and dissolve.

4. Before finishing this method, drain the liquid and dry only the outer part of the ear with a piece of toilet paper, cotton ball, cotton towel or, cotton swab.

PROFESSIONAL SERVICES TO CONSIDER

Previously, it has been stated that you can use homemade remedies for your ears, but nothing beats having a medical professional do the job for you. These practices are often done when you are suffering from serious ear infections or any problem related to your ears, but even if all you want to do is to maintain the cleanliness of your ears, you can try to do this as well.

You may wonder why you would want spend more money if there are plenty of home ear cleaning kits available in the market or even things that you can use that is already available in the comforts of your own home. Well, the reason this may be a better option for you is that a professional knows the best thing to do for you, and having it done by someone who is trained to do this job will pose less of a risk.

Homemade remedies or store-bought remedies can be done, but you MUST follow the instructions very carefully since the eardrum is an extremely sensitive organ, so if you're afraid of taking that risk or if you describe yourself as clumsy, spending a little extra cash will be worth it.

Also, not only is choosing to do this a lot safer, professional services are most likely scientifically proven to clean your ears while doing little to no harm to your ears as it has been tested by doctors. So, you may be wondering what type of ear cleaning services might best fit you.

MICROSUCTION

This is known to be one of the safest forms of earwax removal as it does not use any liquids to remove the debris stuck in your ears. In this method, a vacuum is inserted inside ones ear to gently suction out and extract any excess buildup in the ear. This is done by a medical professional and is a very quick process. This is done whenever a patient feels pain due to the extra earwax that may have been stuck.

IRRIGATION

This was mentioned earlier, but this is also part of the services done by a professional. In this method, a long device made for this very purpose is used and it sprays out water with a slight amount pressure and is put near the entrance of your ear. The gentle rush of water will loosen the earwax and let it naturally drain out of your ear. This procedure is totally safe; some people even find that it is a pleasant experience (sometimes ticklish.)

ALL ABOUT EAR WAX CANDLES

Stated before were methods done by most health care professionals, but now we're going to talk about a method that has been done for a very long time. It can be traced back to the Ancient Greece era. This procedure is used by Chinese, Egyptians and also, Native Americans.

Recently, it has gained popularity once again. Plenty of people on social media sites have been seen with a candle and a plate placed by their ears. It may look funny and you may be curious about what on earth are they doing. Well, this method is what you call "Ear Candling."

WHAT IS EAR CANDLING?

Ear candling, ear coning, or thermal-auricular therapy is an age-old method and was used to balance out the energy within the body of the person trying this technique. This practice starts off with a specially designed candle usually made from unbleached linen or cotton soaked in beeswax.

The materials used for ear candling are generally safe. Most manufacturers use organic and natural products in making these candles, but it is also very important to know where you get these special candles from because there are also plenty of fake and off brand versions of these products. Some are not made with natural ingredients and can be extremely toxic especially since it is used internally. Some people still buy them though because these are sold cheaper in the markets compared to the legitimate ones.

This cloth (usually coated with beeswax, herbs and even honey) is rolled into a long tube and is then inserted into the air canal. After this, the tip of the candle is lit with a small candle flame.

The procedure ends with the leftover burnt cotton being soaked with an amount of water enough to kill the fire then, and then pushing a stick through the remaining tiny piece where the entire residue is left, which includes the earwax and some of the beeswax from the used candle and also a few bits of ashes.

Now, how can this specifically lit candle, really clean and empty out your ears from ear wax? Well, it is said that as the smoke enters your ear canal, it softens and loosens the build-up of impacted cerumen.

Also, as the smoke goes inside the ear, the smoke reacts with and dissolves impurities and dirt that have been constantly building up in your ear. They are converted into gas and go up to the unburned portion of the candle. This is an ancient technique, but has been gaining popularity once again in recent years.

DOES IT WORK?

Now that we have tackled how many practitioners claim it works, it's time to get into whether it is actually scientifically proven? So, it claims to remove impurities in the ear by removing by debris or specs of dirt that may be lodged in your ear. As a result, the likelihood of impacted ear and infections is reduced.

The same mechanism that allows it to clear the canal is also said to help provide relief from or prevent other ear or sinus related complications.

Many of those who have tried this would start the procedure with a congested nose and come out with clear nasal passages.

Not only has that, these people even claimed that this is effective when it comes to relieving stress. However, doctors and scientists alike have stated that the effectiveness of ear candling is backed by little to no evidence. There is not enough scientific evidence or data to that it does work. This is because of the lack of studies conducted about this practice. The FDA (Food and Drug Administration) has forbidden the use of these candles due to the lack of evidence that it is safe and that it actually works.

One of the reasons why people still can have access and do ear candling is that it is labelled to be "for entertainment and leisure purposes only", doctors have said that for the procedure of ear candling to work, it has to be very powerful (the vacuuming effect of the ear candle) to get all of the earwax out from the ear, so powerful that it is impossible for the eardrum not to rupture. There have been many reports about injury related to ear candling. These include accidents such as burns, punctured ear drums and, clogged candle wax in the ear canal that require to be removed surgically. Of course, this has been done by people who have little to no knowledge about ear candling.

As said earlier, ears—namely the eardrum—is highly sensitive. Always have someone who knows what they're doing do the work for you. Paying a little bit more money is always better than risking your overall safety.

While this method does pose some risks depending on whoever is doing this (as most accidents from this is done in unprofessional environments and the usage of cheap and low-quality products) ear candling also has its benefits! It is a form of therapy, and plenty of people who have tried it have had a soothing and relaxing experience. The relaxing feeling is from the herbs and leaves such as chamomile and sage in the ear candle.

This method has been used in spiritual cleansing and was used to balancing the energy in the body. It is used in certain rituals and ceremonies. This method is focused on having you feel calm, renewed, and stress-free! It is comparable to having a traditional type of massage or being in a meditative state. Doing this is described as having your ear massaged by the warm air emitted by the candle.

This practice also balances the sinus and the ears. Since this method isn't supported by much scientific evidence, this is not the total alternative to ear cleaning methods prescribed by your doctor, but that does not mean it doesn't work for other people. Plenty have claimed that their sense of hearing and their sense of smell has enhanced greatly after the procedure. It seems like it could be worth a shot

No ear is the same, and ear candling may or may not work for you. You may go ahead and try it and see if it works, but always prioritize your safety and always have someone who is skilled on this type of thing to do it for you! Never ever attempt to do this without adequate research, knowledge, and practice.

But since you have now delved in the how ear candling works, by this point you have probably made a decision if you would like to try it. You can go ahead see for yourself if it can alleviate any of the symptoms you may be feeling.

A SHORT GUIDE TO USING EAR WAX CANDLES

Ear wax candling is becoming the staple in earwax removal although it has yet to be established as one with the use of scientific data. Ear wax candling also doesn't solve the problem of curing any ear complications that relate to wax (such as infections, pain and the likes). However, ear candling helps keep and the movement or flow of earwax from the inner ear, middle ear and out to the outer ear. This can provide tremendous relief for those with

Ear candling can be a great experience and can work depending on the skill of the practitioner. As long as you're seeking services from people who know exactly what they're doing, you're going to be fine.

If you want in on how it's done, this guide will give you exactly that.

Before starting this method, make sure that you are using the right and proper sized ear candle for your ear, many have claimed that this have not worked for them and this is because of the poor fit of the candle. All of us obviously have different sized ears and that is why many ear candling practitioners have come up with a tapered tip that can be trimmed, making it much easier for any sudden adjustment.

Next, decide whether you want to sit or to lie down. Your head should be in a 60 degree angle. Either of the two positions will work as long as you are positioned in the right angle. Just pick what you think is most relaxing and comfortable for your taste. Most people like laying down for a more therapeutic feel. If you worry about the wax being blocked, keep in mind that cases like this rarely happens and is usually because people did not try to follow the instructions given accurately.

The procedure starts off with the cone-like paper that has been spiraled and is then poked through a plate. (Preferably an aluminum material, paper plates or plastic plates will most often, burn). This plate acts as a protection or barrier for your hair and also your skin (the back of your ear, face and also, neck).

Now, the tip of the candle is placed inside the ear canal by the client to know if it fits very comfortably and is in the right and proper position while the other tip is lit with fire. The tip that has been burnt out to ashes is cut off every now and then and is then doused in water.

Most people who try this out find this the most pleasurable and relaxing because of the crackling sound the burning candle produces. Once the paper candle is short in length or has reached a mark (usually colored red) it means that it is ready to be removed and the process is finally over!

The practitioner ear will usually show the earwax that has been collected through the ear candling process by poking through the candle with a thick stick or by simply unrolling the candle. It is worth a try, and if the process has been effective on you, you'll see how satisfying it is to see all the excess wax on the candle.

CONCLUSION

Our ears, just like any other body parts, play such a big role in our everyday routine. Our body can be quite an amazing system because it works just how it should be, considering what we have to undergo every single day.

Our body basically to adapt to certain conditions in order to survive. But even if it is a fascinating system, we have to give great care to it in order to maximize its abilities and prolong the usage of these parts. The glands in our body secrete certain things for a reason, and one great example is the main topic of the book you are reading right now and it is of course, earwax.

Although earwax is good for you, too much of this can still cause complications that can result to unhygienic outcomes. At a young age we are taught to follow certain routines regularly in order to maintain cleanliness, including cleaning your ears.

Thanks to the advancements done by professionals through thorough researching, we are able to learn more about how to properly give maintenance to the body parts that we have. Sometimes, the discomfort we feel in our ears may not be due to earwax and cleaning may not be the solution for this. Be sure on what the cause of what you are feeling in your ear before doing anything to it.

There are plenty of methods that you can use to clean your ears. There are home remedies that will softly clean your ears without having the risk of damaging your eardrum or causing small abrasions inside your ear. There are also plenty of methods that have been proven to be safe and effective, and a doctor will be able to identify what kind of professional service may be appropriate for your ears.

But even if you use these home remedies for cleaning your ears, you must be careful. You must follow the instructions precisely as it still poses risks. If you want to clean your ears but is not willing to do it all by yourself, seeing a medical professional is the way to go.